MY PERSONAL BATTLE WITH HEART DISEASE

THE HEREDITARY FACTOR

BY

DAVD JAMES ZOPPI

Contents

Preface

My life was going along pretty much like everyone else that I knew. I went to college, graduated and got married and had a child, divorced and married again. In that time, I found a career working with people with disabilities and loved my job. For many years I worked providing employment training and support to people with disabilities in my community. I also work occasionally as a musician performing with my band.

Yes, life was going along just fine until I suffered a heart attack in 2013. I thought perhaps I lifted something too heavy and waited to seek help, which caused heart damage. Well, my world came crashing down around me, and my life and future were uncertain. After I recovered, I had a defibrillator implanted in 2014 and went along for about four years until a stress test revealed two more blockages. It was thought I might need stents, but later determined that I needed double bypass surgery. How could this be? "I asked myself." My cholesterol was 97 and my triglycerides were 143, and yet here I was in the hospital facing surgery.

This is my personal journey battling heart disease and the heredity factor associated with it. I will share my personal story with you to help make clear why sometimes you can be doing everything supposedly right and still face problems and adversity. It is my hope that this book and the information contained herein will help others who are perhaps facing similar problems and/or situations.

"My incisions have become my battle scars reflecting my ongoing fight against an opponent I have come to know as heart disease." David James Zoppi

CHAPTER 1

My Heart Attack

As I was growing up, I never dreamed that anything bad could happen to me like getting a heart attack. Besides, those thing happen to other people and not me, because I thought I was indestructible. Still, I was never obese, I never ate crazy and ate pretty much the way other children, teens and adults ate when I was growing up. In 1977, my mother Elaine Lindsley was diagnosed with Addison's disease which is a disease that attacks the adrenal glands. Shorty afterword's, she had a heart attack and needed quadruple bypass surgery. Then, in 2001, my mother had Aorta repair surgery. She first went to a Doctor in her own state who told her to "Get her affairs in order." After hearing that, she decided to get a second opinion and ended-up going to a hospital in Texas to have the surgery done by one of the best surgeons for this type of surgery. She pulled through the surgery fine and then lived for many years until passing away in May of 2014. Although my mother didn't exercise, she never ate a poor diet and still struggled with heart disease for many years.

Up until the time I had my heart attack, I never ate a diet any different from what my family or friends typically ate, and I was not obese and exercised regularly. I also always prided myself for not having to take any medications at the time before my heart attack, so I thought I was fine. What reinforced this belief was a physical I had one year before my heart attack. Everything checked out fine, *except* for one thing. I received a call from the doctor's office telling me that my cholesterol was high and to get it re-tested. Instead of having it re-tested, I ignored the plea from my doctor's office and dismissed the news and went about my life as though nothing was wrong. This was my *first* mistake, not listening to the advice of my doctor to get my cholesterol retested.   A year later, I had my first heart attack.

At the time I had my first heart attack, I was working in my job as an employment specialist with people with disabilities in the community. I did this job for over fifteen years and enjoyed my work very much. However, I felt tired and listless and felt like something was wrong, but I couldn't quite put my finger on the problem. Unknown to me, the problem was with my heart and I was about to make my second mistake.

In early June of 2013, I woke-up in a cold sweat and remember telling my wife, "Oh my God, I think I had a heart attack."   Instead of acting on that assumption, I got myself together and then somehow convinced myself that the discomfort I felt was from something I lifted the day before because the pain was emanating from my *back* and *not* from my chest, and I had no shortness of breath. Well, the discomfort went away and I was able to go on until August 4th, 2013 which was the day I suffered my second heart attack. I was stubborn and still convinced that the pain I felt was from lifting something heavy because the pain was in my *back* and was not in my chest which was another mistake I made because I *assumed* the pain was something other than a heart attack. When the pain got to be too much, I decided to call my doctor and the physician on call told me it sounded like I was having a heart attack a to get to the emergency room right away.

When I arrived at the local hospital the doctor did an EKG and it was determined that I was having a heart attack. I was then transported to a city hospital. When I arrived the ambulance staff brought me to the operating room where the surgeon was waiting. At that time, he determined that bypass surgery was not needed. He made in incision in my leg to enter through the groin area and placed 3 stents in my arteries. While looking at my heart during the process of placing stents in my arteries, it was determined that I had suffered heart damage from my heart attack, probably because I waited too long to seek medical treatment.

The doctor also made an incision in my left leg and inserted a balloon pump. Basically, the way it was explained to me was that the balloon pump rests near the heart and pumps like a heart to assist the heart with pumping if the heart is deemed too weak initially after a heart attack. It took a while to get used to, because it felt weird having something beating inside your body along with your heart. Although I only had the balloon pump inside of me for about three days, it felt like an eternity.

After the doctor placed the stents and inserted the balloon pump inside of me, I was brought up to the ICU to recover. I had about five nurses in my room inserting IV's and preparing me. After that, I tried to rest the first night and would spend about three days in bed before being allowed to get of bed and into a chair. While flat on my back I had time to ponder the future, while perplexed as to why I was even in the hospital in the first place. Even a nurse who walked by my room, stuck her head inside my room and said, "Sir, you look too good to be in here." That's what I thought too, but heart attacks don't care how you look, or if you exercise or eat right if your body is producing bad cholesterol naturally, as mine was.

By the third day I was able to get out of bed and sit in a chair, which I did as much as possible. Sitting in a chair and getting away from the bed allowed me to put myself in a different frame of mind and mood and helped me to focus on healing and recovery. On the third day, I was also able to receive visitors from friends and relatives. I also received a visit from the hospital administration, the financial department. The lady who visited me discussed ways to help me to pay for my medical expense, including filing for social security disability and Medicaid; which I did as soon as I got home from the hospital. Without Medicaid and assistance from Social Services, I would have had to pay an $85,000 hospital bill and a $6,000 bill for the stent procedure.

When the fourth day came, I was brought up to a private room from the ICU. I felt good but was constipated from inactivity, and tried stool softeners and prune juice and nothing worked. So, I just toughed it out and knew that in time once I started walking, I would go. My cousin from Virginia is a doctor and administrator told me that, "Once you start moving again, it will get things moving along inside of you and you will go again." Fortunately, not long after I left the hospital, my primary care physician recommended a laxative that worked great and is the laxative that I have used ever since.

Once I was moved from the ICU to a private room, a number of nurses began to put the fear of God into me, and I owe each of them my gratitude. When I was recovering, I remember the first nurse came into my room to talk to me about the importance of taking my meds and not forgetting to take them. She also told me not to lift anything heavy or to shovel. I was told that if I shovel snow that I could essentially drop dead. I listened to and took her advice.

The second nurse that spoke to me told also told me the importance of taking my medications. He also told me how many people return to the hospital because they ignored taking their medications. I assured him that I would take all medications as prescribed. He was happy to hear that I would stick to the program and follow the doctor's orders.

The third nurse told me that I should not allow my weight to go above 2 pounds a day or five pounds a week, or else I would risk getting congestive heart failure. I didn't like the way that sounded and stayed the course with my diet upon leaving the hospital and lost twenty-five pounds and bottomed-out at a target weight of one-hundred thirty eight pounds. He also gave me a list of the medications that I would need to take and went over when to take them. He also stressed the importance of taking all medications as prescribed. However, the nurse told me that sometimes people do forget to take their medications. So, he said that, "If you can't remember if you took your medications, then do not take them for that day."

Upon discharge, I was given a list of instructions and materials to read along with dietary suggestions to follow. I only wish I know then what I know now about Trans fats, saturated fats and sodium. Still, I lost the weight, worked hard to get into great shape and did my best to keep well and to stay well. Along with the discharge papers were instructions for follow-ups with my cardiologist and my primary care physician.

A few weeks after discharge, I went for a follow-up with my cardiologist. When I was called into the examination room the doctor listened to my heart and told me everything sounded good. Then, he told me that he needed to discuss a few things with me. I knew it wasn't going to be good, but whatever the news would be, I realized that I needed to hear it. The doctor told me that I would be unable to go back to working with people with disabilities, and also told me that I would need to have a defibrillator implanted because my hearts ability to pump blood out was compromised due to a low ejection fraction of only fifteen percent at the time.

When I was told that I could not return to work, my world came crashing down. For years I went to college, walked college campuses in rain, sleet, snow and heat and worked so hard to get my master's degree and find a job I loved, all to see it come to an end. Being told that I needed surgery to have a defibrillator implanted in my body further complicated my life. I didn't want any of this, it was like a bad dream. I thought perhaps if I closed my eyes and opened them again that it would all go away and I could return to my regular life, but unfortunately, it was all too real. Facing life without employment was very scary prospect. However, once I was able to get the help I needed from Social Security and from Social Services, I was able to slowly put some of the pieces of my life back together and move forward. I was used to helping others in my work, but now I had to depend on the help of others myself, since my heart condition classified me as being totally and permanently disabled.

CHAPTER 2

Cardiac Rehabilitation

To regain my life, I needed to regain my independence. It was a slow process at first, and started with ten minutes of walking in the morning the first week after returning home from the hospital. Then, I was walking fifteen to twenty minutes in the morning and in the evening the second week after getting out of the hospital. Finally, I was walking thirty minutes a day prior to starting cardiac rehabilitation. I remember the first time I started walking after leaving the hospital that I couldn't even feel my heart beating in my chest. It was though there was not even a heart there, no presence, nothing at all. However, in time as I started walking more, my heart got stronger and I could feel it beating and pumping blood.

A number of weeks later I started cardiac rehabilitation at a local hospital. I didn't know what to expect and had no idea what I would be able to do once I started, and what I could do in the future.   When I entered the cardiac rehabilitation room I saw many elderly men and women who had suffered heart attacks, and a few people who were closer to my age as well. A few people looked at me as though I didn't belong there, but there were many others who joined cardiac rehabilitation who were very close to my age. A heart attack knows does not recognize age or how well you eat if there are other factors at work, such as the *hereditary factor.*

The heart attack had taken many things away from me in an instant. I was unable to return to my job and many aspects of my life that I knew and was familiar with, but now I had a chance to regain a level of independence to get me back into doing many of the things I did before. I realized that I had two choices. I could turn my back on heart disease and get lost in a pool of emotion, or I could fight and take heart disease head-on. I chose to take heart disease head-on and to fight.

Once I started my first session at cardiac rehabilitation, the nurse had me get on the scale. I was 138 pounds at the time, and had lost about 20 - 25 pounds since my heart attack. After getting weighed, contacts were taped to my chest to monitor my heart, and I was then directed to the treadmill. I started walking on the treadmill for twelve minutes, then after that I used the exercise bike for 12 minutes, and finally I used a machine that worked my arms for 12 minutes. So, at twelve minute intervals I was doing thirty-six minutes of activity at cardiac rehab.

The months passed quickly, but during that time I never did anything on my own activity-wise other than what I did in cardiac rehabilitation. If I wanted to walk on the days that I didn't have cardiac rehabilitation I asked if that was acceptable. I always checked and asked questions to make sure that I was never going too much or too little. I realized that asking lots of questions was important so that I could eventually devise my own exercise plan to keep me fit and well.

As time went on, I got stronger and was able to learn how much I could do. I was told that I could even do resistance band training and lift up to 10 pounds at the time. I always hurt myself lifting, so I stayed away from the 10 pound weights and stuck to the treadmill and resistance band training. I was told basically that I could do these activities to tolerance. So, after leaving cardiac rehabilitation three months later, I joined a gym and was able to continue using a treadmill and bike. In time, my wife bought a treadmill for me for the home and I was able to use that instead of going to the gym. I continued my resistance band training and also did isometrics, yoga, Tai Chi and also started taking karate online and working toward getting my back belt.

When I entered cardiac rehabilitation I was so frightened of all the things that I might not be able to do or to do again. However, the staff at cardiac rehabilitation taught me and showed me all the things that I *could* do! In time, I was doing activities I never dreamed I would be doing, and exceeding all of my expectations. The cardiac rehabilitation staff replaced my fear with hope and optimism for the future. They helped me to take back my life and regain my independence and gave me a new outlook on life and for the future.

CHAPTER 3

Maintaining a Healthy Diet

It has been said that "diet and exercise go hand-in-hand." Well, it's true, a healthy diet and exercise go a long way in managing heart disease. You can look at a label title in the market and see words like "*Organic*" or "*Healthy*" or "*Vegan*" but then take a look at the nutritional information. You would be surprised to learn that many products with a label saying "*Organic*" or "*Healthy*" or "*Vegan*" had high amounts of sodium, Trans fats and/or saturated fats. You really need to read the labels and count your daily sodium, Trans fat and saturated fat intake. You need to make an appointment to consult with a dietitian to ask questions about planning meals and learn how to structure your meals and make healthy choices.

Before my heart attack I exercised and didn't eat a lot of junk foods, but I also did not take all of the risk factors into consideration, such as heredity.   Diet and exercise was not enough in my case, and not being on cholesterol medication and ignoring the one risk factor that posed a threat to my health almost cost me my life, which is the **hereditary factor**. Do not just *assume* that your diet is sufficient and that you exercise enough; especially if you have a family history or the risk factors associated with a particular disease or condition.

After my heart attack I was given a list of meals that I could eat. One of the meals that were listed was a popular *healthy* frozen dinner. Well, because it was on the list, I thought it would be fine. However, I was unaware of the high sodium content. So, just because a label suggests that you are making a healthy selection YOU must investigate further. Check the sodium, the Trans fats and saturated fats and ask your dietitian what the daily allowances are for you for each of these. Ask about bread selections and what best choices are such as whole wheat versus whole grain choices for instance.

After my heart attack I cut out and limited many foods. I cut caffeine and fast foods from my diet, limited salt intake and fruit juices kept my weight within two pounds day and five pounds a week because of the threat of getting congestive heart failure. I also limited my sugar intake and used a sugar substitute instead. However, I continued to eat butter which was 50% less fat and low sodium cheese. I also ate the *healthy* frozen dinners which were on the list of foods the hospital gave me, not knowing how high in sodium they were at the time.

So, as much as I thought I was doing right, I was still doing a lot of things wrong. I should have been reading labels and taking sodium, trans and saturated fats into account and writing down the content of each of those so that I stayed within 2,000MG of sodium or less daily. I would see an apple pie and think to myself, "Wow, its sugar free, so it must be alright for me to eat it." Unfortunately, I failed to look at the sodium content. Or, I would go to a buffet with my wife and take a spoonful of Macaroni and Cheese, not realizing that even though I was taking a small portion, that things like cheese, dairy and butter were not doing my heart any good. Therefore, that is why it is so important to educate yourself, ask questions and also to consult with a dietitian. It is very easy to fall back into old habits or to make-up your own rules as you go along, "Well, it's alright if I have a little bit of that macaroni, a few French fries and one chicken finger from the Chinese buffet *this time*." Problem is that pretty soon, you start applying that reasoning all the time, and start taking a little bit of this and a little bit of that. Well, a little bit of this and a little bit of that all adds up and can create more problems down the road.

A healthy turkey sandwich with whole grain bread can actually turn out to be not so healthy if we choose a turkey high in sodium, or drench it in dressing high in fat and sodium and use lots of cheese for instance. It's not just what we eat, but how we eat it that can make it healthy or unhealthy for consumption. For instance, I use lots of substitutes for the foods I can't eat and for spices. Instead of salt, I use a salt substitute made-up of herbs which is great for meals and on sandwiches. For cheese slices, I now use a Tofu cheese instead of regular cheese which I out on my sandwiches. I also use hummus instead of cheese which adds lot of flavor to my sandwiches.

There are a variety of protein sources which I use that are great alternatives. *Quinoa* is known mainly for its edible seeds and is very nutritious, contains lots of fiber, iron, manganese and magnesium. *Soy* is a great protein and an excellent substitute for those who are on a vegan diet. *Ezekiel Bread* is generally made from sprouted grains, but can be made by combining lentils, wheat, beans, barley, millet, and spelt and then placed into a bowl and formed into bread. **Rice and Beans** is a very easy and inexpensive vegan dish to make and is a great source of protein. When you substitute chick peas or lentils for beans, you have a great vegan dish full of carbs and protein! A *Peanut Butter Sandwich* is easy to make and is a great choice which contains lots of healthy fats also contains amino acids. *Hummus and Pita -* Hummus is a spread or dip made from cooked, mashed chickpeas or other types of beans and are then blended with lemon juice, salt and garlic, tahini and olive oil. In the Middle East it is very popular. Chickpeas amino acids are similar to that of most legumes. So hummus and Pita are an excellent meal and great source of lysine as well.

When consulting with my dietitian, she told me that healthful diet typically contains less than five grams of saturated fat. Most of *saturated fat* comes from animal products such as pork, poultry with skin, lamb, beef, cheese, cream, butter and additional dairy products as well as those created from whole and 2 percent milk. All of these foods also consist of dietary cholesterol. For those who need to lower their cholesterol, it is suggested to *reduce saturated fat to no more than 5 to 6 percent of total daily calories.*

Unsaturated fat such as polyunsaturated and monounsaturated fats are the two unsaturated fats. These are found primarily in fish such as herring, trout, salmon and olives, walnuts, avocados and vegetable oils such consisting of corn, olive, safflower, canola, soybean, and sunflower as well. Polyunsaturated and monounsaturated fats may help improve cholesterol in the blood utilized to replace saturated and *trans* fats.

Trans fats (or *trans* fatty acids) adds hydrogen to liquid vegetable oils to make them more solid. *Trans* fats are also known as "partially hydrogenated oils." These *Trans* fats in many baked goods as well as fried foods such as cookies and crackers, pizza dough, pastries and pie crust. These *Trans* fats increase bad (LDL) cholesterol levels and lower your good (HDL) cholesterol levels. It is these changes which can be attributed with a higher risk of heart disease.

I also like to use vegan substitutes as well. For pizza, I choose a whole wheat pita bread with flax and use a teaspoon of olive oil and coat the top of the pita bread. Then, I place a teaspoon of hummus on top of the pita bread in the middle and spread it around the top. Next, I use a no salt spaghetti sauce and spread that around the top of the pita bread. Finally, I use a handful of chick peas which I sprinkle over the top of the pita bread and place it on a small baking sheet and put it into the toaster oven. The pita bread pizza is allowed to bake for 12 minutes at 325 - 350 degrees.

In the meantime, I prepare a veggie burger. Some can be microwaved and others can be warmed-up in a frying pan with a little olive oil. Just check the label to determine the salt content. Coordinate the time it takes to cook your veggie burger with the time it will take for your pita bread pizza to finish baking. Some veggie burgers take about 2 minutes or less in the microwave while others could take longer if a frying pan is used; perhaps up to 15 minutes. Once the pita bread pizza is finished baking, grab an oven glove and remove the pizza and baking sheet pan from the oven and then remove the cooked veggie burger. Then, dice the veggie burger and distribute it evenly across the top of the pita bread pizza. If you wish, you can add more sauce and microwave it for 15 - 20 seconds. Otherwise, you're pita bread pizza is done and ready to be eaten!

Health food stores are also a great place to find heart healthy soups, snacks and more. Remember, just because a label says *organic* or *healthy* doesn't mean that it is. You need to READ THE LABEL!!! I can't begin to tell you how many times I've seen labels like this, only to learn that the sodium content was extremely high. I searched for a soup low in sodium for many months after my heart attack, but to no avail. Most of the soup sodium content I found was extremely high. It wasn't until I checked out a health food store and the health food isles in the market that I discovered a minestrone soup with no sodium. Also, if you like making your soups homemade, you can also buy the ingredients and make the soup yourself. When you make your own meals, YOU control the amount of sodium, if any, that you put into your food.

If you're like me, then you have a sweet tooth. Well, sodium, butter and more can be in sweets, so once again, you must read those labels. There are fruit preserves on the market that contain no fats and no sodium that go perfect on whole grain bread! If you like crunchy snacks, then there are lots of great choices such as:

- Bell pepper slices
- Zucchini or cucumber
- Pears and apples
- Seeds and nuts
- Roasted chickpeas
- Celery sticks and Carrot
- Popcorn
- Rice cakes and whole-grain crackers
- Seeds and nuts
- Roasted chickpeas
- Broccoli and cauliflower

What you drink is as important as what you eat, so it is essential to re-evaluate beverages. For instance, you can drink:

- Tea or coffee (Unsweetened or use an artificial sweetener)
- Decaf. Coffee or decaf. Green tea.
- Sparkling or plain water
- A small glass of 100% fruit juice
- Plain Soymilk or fat-free milk
- Mixed vegetable juice or Low-sodium tomato

Snacks not only need to be wholesome, but they need to be satisfying as well!

Some snacks that curb your hunger are:

- Whole-grain toast with peanut or almond butter
- Cherry tomatoes with hummus
- Low-fat or fat-free cheese
- Plain low-fat or fat-free yogurt (An awesome pairing with fruit!)
- Fruit smoothie
- Hummus with Cherry tomatoes
- Whole-grain crackers
- Whole-grain toast with almond butter or peanut butter
- Whole-grain bread with olive oil

Also, these snacks are great to satisfy that sweet tooth:

- Banana-nut bread (watch portion)
- Angel food cake (watch portion)
- Raisins, dates, figs and other unsweetened dried fruits
- Fresh fruit salad
- Canned fruit (in natural juice or light syrup)
- Baked apple
- Frozen grapes

Trans fats, saturated fats, daily recommended sodium intake and more can be confusing. Unfortunately, I had to learn by trial and error, but I learned and I'm using the knowledge I learned to help myself and to help others. Eating low-fat, low-sodium and low sugar can be an adventure! For instance, you can experiment and have fun with food choices. For instance, you might try buying a cook book on Mediterranean cooking and explore all of the possibilities. When I started exploring a Mediterranean diet, I found a whole new world of options. From soups to salads, poultry to fish and more, I discovered many great meal ideas!

Being a heart patient even though I follow a strict diet, I never feel like I'm giving up anything or losing out on anything. Since I've given up fast foods I've left all that fat and grease and sodium behind and have started on a life-long journey of healthful eating. I am aware of my sodium, trans fat and saturated fat intake and now have a good handle on my diet. Food and eating have become fun again since I have started cooking my own meals and exploring healthy alternatives and choices and more!

CHAPTER 4

Exercise

It has been said that, "Diet and exercise go hand-in-hand." This is very true, and exercise under the direction of a cardiac rehabilitation program and your doctor are very important. As I stated, I never started an exercise program or did any kind of exercise before first consulting with my physician. I also consulted with cardiac rehabilitation and my cardiac surgeon before trying any new exercises or endeavors. ***So, before starting any kind of exercise, consult first with your physician!***

After cardiac rehabilitation, I continued the exercise routine established by cardiac rehabilitation by joining a fitness club. At the fitness club, I did the same routine that I was instructed to do at cardiac rehabilitation until we bought a treadmill for the home. I also mixed it up a bit during the warm-weather months. I remember the first time I walked outside on the walking trail for thirty minutes. I remembered the nurse telling me how the heart likes oxygen, so I tried to walk outside on days that were not rainy or humid during the summer months. I remember the day when I had realized after a thirty minute walk that I breathed in and out entirely through my nose. At that point, I realized that I was reaching a level of cardiac fitness that I could be proud of, and eventually my heart rate reached 50 beats per minutes, the level of an athlete.

In time, I started considering getting my black belt in karate online. I asked myself if I could I do this. The more I studied the karate videos in the online program, the more convinced I was that I *could* undertake this challenge and life-long dream. I consulted with my doctor and told him that basically the movements were like choreographed dance movements. The doctor approved my request to take Karate lessons online and I started immediately!

The initial belts were easy, but they got harder as I went along. Kicking routines and Kata's (which are individual training exercises) tested my cardiovascular fitness, but I did fine. In time, I worked up from my white belt to a blue belt in karate. I also started doing Thai Chi and using resistance cables for upper-body strength.

I remember the staff at cardiac rehabilitation telling me that I could do the resistance cable exercises to tolerance. So, in my case, I was able to work up to about 30-35 reps for each exercise that I did, and did 3 sets of each exercise. I basically did *biceps and back* on Mondays and Thursdays, *triceps and shoulders* on Tuesdays and Fridays, and *legs and chest* on Wednesdays and Saturdays. I did leg stretching exercises daily that consisted of leg extensions, squats and lunges without any kind of weights, and thirty to thirty-six minutes on the treadmill daily.

With resistance band training, I experimented with different exercises and any exercises that were too strenuous or put too much strain on me I omitted. For instance, I wrapped one of my resistance bands around bed post and did seated cable rows, only to feel muscular strain in my chest. Well, the sensation of a strained chest made it impossible for me to tell if I was having another heart attack, or if it was just muscular strain, which prompted me to make a visit to the emergency room at the hospital. I was checked out and it was decided that I had pulled a muscle and that it was *not* a heart attack.

This experience had taught me not to over-do it and to stick with a program of exercise that was beneficial and not harmful or hurtful to me. Before my heart attack I was bodybuilding and lifting weights. I would always manage to strain myself and have to start over again. It reminds me of the story I was told in my youth of the little boy who had a bucket and filled his bucket by collecting marbles from the ground. His bucket was almost full when all at once, he stumbled on a stone and all of the marbles fell out of the bucket. The boy then proceeded to start over again putting picking up marbles and putting them back into the bucket.

Well, as patient I was getting tired of getting injured and having to start over again and again and again. So, I changed my approach to exercise. I knew that in addition to getting injured when body building, I was also getting older. So, I chose to substitute body building with resistance band training and isometric training by *simulating weight training movements* using a kind of strength training in which the joint angle and muscle length remain constant during contraction. I chose the treadmill and walking outside in place of biking and running. Also, any exercise or activity which caused me pain or discomfort I omitted from my workouts.

After a time, I also incorporated yoga into my workouts. Yoga got its start in ancient India, and uses mental, spiritual and physical disciplines or practices which originated in ancient India. Like resistance band training, I chose and used the exercises that worked for me and did not cause me pain or discomfort. If you chose not to do yoga on your own, you can always sign-up for classes, but remember *always* to get permission from your physician prior to starting *any* kind of exercise training on your own or before starting classes or joining a gym. Also, stay within the parameters set by your doctor and adhere to all restrictions your doctor tells you to follow.

After completing three months of cardiac rehabilitation and asking the cardiac rehabilitation staff what exercises I could and could not do and how much I could do, I was able to begin exploring different types of exercise. I changed-up my workouts to keep them more interesting, fresh and exciting as well and over time had developed a level of muscle strength and toning as well as outstanding cardiac level of fitness that I was proud of. However, I did have some restrictions.

I was told that if I worked out with dumbells that I should limit the weight to ten pounds. I was informed that I had no limits on stairs, but I still use common sense when approaching stairs. I will generally go half-way up a flight of stairs, wait and then proceed the rest of the way. If I am outside or faced with climbing a long flight of stairs, then I will go as far as I can comfortably, wait and then do a little bit more and if people are behind me, then I just tell then to go around me. I also have to be careful of really humid days and also days that are excessively cold.

I recently went on a vacation this past summer with family to Washington, New York City and Philadelphia and it was very humid when we visited Philadelphia. One of the places I wanted to see was the art museum steps where the movie "*Rocky III*" was filmed to see the "Rocky Statue." I remember that in the movie, the "Rocky Statue" was located at the top of a long flight of stairs. I pondered how I would climb the stairs, but once I arrived to my surprise, I could see that statue had been moved to the lower street-level for people to come and take pictures with the statue.

On another occasion I went to Carnegie Hall to hear a performance of my wife's Uncle's music. When we were in the taxi, the taxi got stuck in traffic and we had to walk the rest of the way which was about three or four blocks. Fortunately, it was not too cold but still cold enough. However, getting out of a taxi and walking out in the winter cold was something that I could do because aerobically I am in excellent condition. However, those are unnecessary risks for others who are *not* in good physical condition. That is why it is absolutely imperative that you follow your doctor's instructions and obey all restrictions.

Yes, I was doing everything I could to stay well between diet and exercise. I watched what I ate and followed all the doctor's orders. It seemed like all was going along fine, until my next office visit. Because of my low ejection fraction which affected my hearts' ability to pump blood out, I had more disappointing news that I would soon face.

CHAPTER 5

Heredity, Adversity and Setbacks

My life seemed to be going along well until my next office visit at the cardiologist. I remember walking into the office of my cardiologist. He listened to my heart and told me it sounded fine. Then, he told me he had some matters of concern to discuss with me. First, he told me that because my heart attack was serious that he thought I should retire from my job working with people with disabilities, which was devastating. I loved working with the disabled and could not imagine my life without my work. The doctor also told me that I would need to have a Defibrillator implanted because my hearts' ejection fraction (ability to pump blood out of the heart) was compromised by my heart attack.

Now, I had to deal with the realization that life had thrown me a curve ball. When this happens, it is not always something that you can change, but must be accepted as just one more thing in life to deal with; it is something that was is unforeseen. My cardiologist gave me a referral to a Doctor who would do additional tests to see if I would need a defibrillator and to discuss the procedure and to show me the type of defibrillator that would be implanted inside me. Since I had stents instead of bypass surgery, I considered myself fortunate. So, I scheduled the appointment with the Doctor for the following week.

The following week, I met with the defibrillator doctor. He sat down across from me and told me about the procedure of implanting a defibrillator. From what I remember, the defibrillator was to be implanted around the left collarbone area and a wire would run down into the heart. The idea of having a wire running down into my heart did not appeal to me. Then, he searched for a defibrillator to show me and found a defibrillator that looked like it had the circumference of a hockey puck or a smoke alarm. I wondered how on earth they would fit and implant something so large inside me because I had such a small frame. I had many questions and many doubts. I kept telling myself that there had to be a better alternative.

When I got home I logged onto my computer and began my research for other options and alternatives. First, I found a vest that is worn under your clothes with a defibrillator woven inside the vest. I thought that this would be the perfect alternative to surgery until I discovered that it was only worn by people temporarily until the actual defibrillator surgery is done. I continued searching the internet until I found an alternative to having a traditional defibrillator implanted. I had found a new defibrillator called the S-ICD. An S-ICD is an implantable cardioverter defibrillator which is also referred to as an ICD which administers a shock if a person suffers cardiac arrest. The same is true if the defibrillator detects a high heart rate it deems dangerous. In contrast to the trans venous ICD which is implanted near the collarbone, the S-ICD is generally implanted on the left side of the chest next adjacent the rib cage. Then, the lead wire is implanted just under the skin above the breastbone, rendering the heart and blood vessels untouched by the lead wire.

Upon visiting the defibrillator doctor I mentioned the S-ICD device to him and asked if he, or one of his associates performed this procedure. Because the procedure was so new and cutting-edge, the doctor told me that there were surgeons taking classes to learn how to perform the procedure. This didn't set well with me. I didn't want someone operating on me who had just learned the procedure. I wanted someone operating on me who *knew* the procedure and had already had some experience performing the procedure. I did some more research and found a surgeon from my city hospital who had performed many of these procedures successfully. I immediately made an appointment to see him.

The following week, I went to see the new defibrillator doctor and he explained the procedure to me. I was really happy because the defibrillator would be implanted under the skin on my left side instead of near my collarbone, and the lead wire would run along my rib cage and up my breast bone with no wires going into my heart. The other thing I really liked was that the defibrillator analyzes a number of heart rhythms before administering a shock and allows you to try to correct a fast heart rate yourself using a vagal technique such as coughing for instance. The only thing the doctor told me which I didn't like was that they needed to stop the heart during surgery to test the device. I told the doctor that I did not want my heart stopped, and to just implant the device without testing it. The doctor agreed and the surgery was schedules for the following month.

My surgery was scheduled for October of 2014. However, I worried about so many things and made myself so sick with worry that I decided to postpone the surgery. This was my first invasive procedure since having my appendix taken out at age three which required anesthesia, so I wanted to make sure I was prepared mentally prepared, because I believe that your mental state, or state of mind is as important as your physical preparedness for surgery.

Well, the month passed quickly and before I knew it, November 17th had arrived, and I went through with the procedure. I remember the doctor doing some preliminary tests the morning of the surgery and telling me that everything looked great! When it was time, I was wheeled down to the operating room. I expected it to be dark and everyone to be wearing their surgical masks. However, to my surprise they had music playing in the operating room and everyone made me feel at ease. I reminded the doctor not to stop the heart and had them give me a doughnut-shaped pillow for my head since I get occasional sleep apnea. I lied down flat on the operating table and then I was given an oxygen mask and a covering over my body. Then, the last thing I remember was the anesthesiologist saying, "Let's get this show in the road."

The next thing I remember was waking-up in the operating room. It was funny because time seemed transient when under anesthetic. It almost seems like you just close your eyes and then wake up and you are not aware of all the time that passed in-between going under the anesthetic and waking up. As I was waking-up I was wheeled to a room where other patients were also recovering. I was then given my medications and asked what I wanted for lunch. After, I was brought down the hall for additional x-rays and then allowed to leave that same day!

When I arrived back home, I sat down on the couch with a pillow and tried to watch television, but quickly realized that perhaps bed was the best place for me to properly recover. I rested in bed on and off for the next three days and walked in the morning and in the evening according to the hospitals instructions, and in the following weeks increased the duration of those walks as instructed. For about ten days, my defibrillator felt like a small ash tray weighing heavily on my side. I didn't know if I would ever get used to it. However, by the eleventh day, when I took a breath, I could feel the defibrillator moving with my diaphragm as I breathed in and out and it was starting to settle-in and feel more like a part of me.

Over the next three years my condition improved dramatically. My ejection fraction went up about 5-10 percent, I was exercising on the treadmill for thirty minutes a day, seven times a week and doing isometrics, resistance band training, yoga and working on getting my back belt in karate. Yes, all was going well, until August of 2017 when I would have to face a new challenge from heart disease.

CHAPTER 6

Returning to the Hospital

It was the month of August of 2017, and I had just reached over my treadmill in my home to close a stubborn window that was stuck and in doing so hurt my shoulder. Well, instead of walking on the treadmill, I decided to walk outside and get some fresh air that day. I walked a short distance and then I felt a dull ache in my shoulders and it started to build-up gradually. I remember a feeling of anxiety come over me, because it was almost the same feeling I had when I had my heart attack, minus the chest pain.

Well, this time I didn't assume anything. I got into my car and informed my wife that I would be going straight to the local hospital. Instead of going to the city hospital, I went to the local town hospital to get checked out since it was the closest. Once I checked-in at the emergency room I was admitted right away and blood samples were taken which included two tests called cardiac marker tests, taken hours apart and the results compared. The emergency room doctor told me that I wasn't having a heart attack, which was a relief. I told the doctor that when I went for a walk that I felt a dull ache building-up in my shoulders, but it went away as soon as I stopped walking. The doctor said that because I felt this ache when I engaged in physical activity that I should schedule a stress test with my cardiologist. This was advice which would prove to save my life.

The following day I scheduled a Nuclear Stress Test with my cardiologist in two weeks. In that two week period up to the time of the appointment I continued to work out on the treadmill, do my resistance band training, isometrics and karate. Sometimes, I would feel the ache in my shoulders while on the treadmill, and other times I would not. On the day of my stress test, once I arrived at the doctor's office a gentleman that I did not recognize called me into the office to take pictures of my heart while I lay flat upon a metal table and I was given a radioactive substance that was injected into my veins. I remember the machine over me taking pictures on my left side, and then working its way in a semi-circular fashion around my chest and stopping at times over my chest to take pictures of my heart. Sometimes, it made me feel anxious, almost claustrophobic when the machine taking the pictures would stop over my chest and move in closer to my chest to take pictures. I was afraid it would crush me which was silly of me to think, but it never got that close.

The entire procedure took about 15 - 20 minutes. Next, I was asked to walk on a treadmill. My heart rhythm and blood pressure were monitored throughout the test. Once again, a radioactive substance was injected into one of my veins. Then, again the special camera scanned my heart and took pictures. After the procedure was over, I went home and waited for the results of the stress test. About two days later I received a call on my cell phone instead of my landline which I thought was strange. I picked up the phone and it was my cardiologist contacting me personally instead of the office staff. He told me that after doing the stress test that a "glitch" was found. I was informed that I would need to schedule a hospital visit to possibly have stents implanted into the arteries of my heart since several did not look like they were getting enough blood. I then scheduled the appointment within two weeks from that time to enter the hospital.

The first time I had a stent procedure was when I had my heart attack in 2013. At that point I had three stents and a heart balloon pump inserted through my leg and positioned inside me to rest near my heart to pump along with my heart to assist it while it got strong again. I remember being in bed flat on my back for about three days, and in that time I swore that I would do everything necessary to stay well and never return to the hospital. I dieted, gave up fast foods, caffeine, watched what I ate and kept my weight within two pounds of my target weight each day and within five pounds a week and exercised regularly and even lost twenty-five to thirty pounds. Yet, here I was once again after all the hard work facing the possibility of yet another heart procedure and additional blockages.

Even after receiving this news, I continued to exercise each day. When the time came to go to the hospital I admitted myself into the hospital and was brought-up to a room where many nurses and other patients were. I was told that if I needed stents that I would just stay in bed eight hours and then be allowed to return home. So, I expected everything to go well so that I get it done and go home. That all sounded great and I was looking forward to getting this stent procedure done and then finding out what caused these additional blockages in the first place.

I remember feeling a wide range of emotions. I felt fear, the *fear* of not knowing what to expect. I felt *frustration* in just having to be there. I also felt *anger* with myself because I blamed myself for having to return to the hospital. I thought I did everything *right*, and yet everything turned out so terribly *wrong*. I had a cholesterol level of around 98 and my triglycerides were 143. So, why did I have to be there in the first place if my numbers were so good? So many unanswered questions that needed to be asked and answered.

After a time, a gentleman came to wheel me down to the room where the stent procedure would be done. The first time it was done when I had my heart attack it was done very quickly and a small monitor was used while the doctor implanted three stents into the arteries of my heart. However, this time the procedure was more involved, more complex and bit scary from a patient prospective. I remember the operating room was well lit and I was freezing and shivering, partly from being cold and partly from the chill of fear taking over me. I remember the kindness of a nurse who bought me a heated towel which she placed over my chest to keep me warm. I was very appreciative and thanked her. I will always remember her thoughtfulness and her kindness.

The next thing I remember was a doctor entering the room that I did not recognize. He was an associate of my cardiologist. I wanted to make sure that my cardiologist would be performing the procedure. His associate reassured me that my cardiologist would be performing the procedure and he was just there to assist. When you see people or things that don't seem right, do not be afraid to question. Do not be afraid of hurting people's feelings or bruising egos. It is your body and you have a right to know who is going to be performing your procedure or operation and what the procedure or operation involves. You also have the right to a second opinion.

After my cardiologists associate entered the operating room, my cardiologist entered a few moments later. I was injected with something made my insides feel briefly flushed with warmth, and then the sensation quickly disappeared. A large monitor screen was positioned on my left which looked like a giant television screen, or big screen TV. It had my name on it at the bottom and was used by the doctors and staff as the procedure was being done. Both of my legs were prepped for the procedure, but only my right leg was used.

My cardiologist made a small incision into the skin of the groin area of my right leg and inserted the probe which would give them a look inside my body to see the arteries of my heart. After exploring with the probe, my cardiologist informed me that I had two new blocked arteries, he told me that he would not be able to do the stent procedure because it was too risky and informed me that I would have to have a double bypass, or open heart surgery. This news was devastating for me. Aside from having a defibrillator implanted, I had not had major surgery since I was three years old when I had my appendix removed. I was then told by the cardiologist and his assistant in the room to take care of this right away and not to wait.

I was then brought back the room I was in before and informed my wife of the news. A short time later, the cardiac surgeon visited me with my cardiologist and told me that his success rate was ninety-eight percent and showed me a diagram of the procedure he would do on a piece of paper.   There was really no time for a second opinion, so I decided to have the cardiac surgeon at the hospital do the surgery. It was a Friday, and the cardiac surgeon told me that he wanted to do the surgery the following Monday, which meant I would have to remain in bed, in the hospital until the surgery on Monday. Well, I was a few pounds underweight and did not want to get weak over the weekend. I also wanted to get myself in the proper mental state. So, against the doctors wishes I told him I would schedule the surgery a week from the following Monday. My cardiologist was not pleased and made me sign waver release before leaving the hospital stating in effect that I was leaving against his wishes.

Each day after until the surgery, I prepared myself mentally and physically. I stayed off my treadmill as the nurse suggested, but went to the mall daily and walked from one end of the mall to the other for thirty minutes each day. I kept utilizing positive self-talk and visualization as well. I kept reminding myself of the doctor's great track record and his success rate and outstanding reputation and kept telling myself that I was in excellent hands. I imagined myself facing my surgery boldly and bravely and then coming out of surgery and getting stronger and better each and every day and successfully navigating the road to recovery. I read books on navy seal mental preparation and reminded myself that I needed to not look at the whole immense picture, but to break it down and take this one step, one challenge at a time.

Well, my decision to postpone my surgery did not sit well with my primary care physician as well. My cardiologist contacted my primary care physician who in turn contacted me. He told me that he was concerned and my cardiologist was concerned as well. I reassured my primary care physician that I would have the surgery scheduled for the following week, and he was relieved to hear this news and accepted it. I guess I was obstinate because heart disease had taken control of my life and taken so much away from me that this time, I was going to take a stand and not let heart disease dictate to me my course of action. I would do want needed to be done, but I was determined to do it on *my* terms, regardless of the risks of waiting and regardless of the advice I received from my doctors. It was a risky and foolish decision, but it was *mine* to make.

The week progressed along and about mid-week I received a call from the cardiac surgeon's office to schedule the surgery which was scheduled for the following Monday at 7am in the morning. The following day, the doctor's office called back and told me that the time had changed from 7am in the morning to 9am in the morning. I was happy that they made it later so that I did not have to get-up too early, but I was still worried about the surgery. The staff I spoke to at the cardiac surgeons office also scheduled a meeting with a nurse the Friday before the surgery to go over the procedure and answer any questions that I might have.

Until the day of the surgery I worried each night, but managed to fall off to sleep, only to awaken one or two hours before my alarm was set to go off, worried and pondering the surgery. Then, my wife would wake up and reassure me that the surgery was common place and routine and not to worry. Although I felt mentally and physically prepared, I still worried. It is a human emotion and I think that that it is perfectly natural. I understood what my wife was saying and used that as part of my positive self-talk. However, it easy for others to reassure us when they themselves do not have to go through the ordeal themselves. No one in the world could understand the fears, worries and apprehensions that I was experiencing better than myself.

When Friday morning arrived, I and my wife traveled to the hospital for the visit with the nurse. When we got to the hospital I announced myself at the front desk and stated that I had an appointment. A few moments later we were greeted by the nurse who brought my wife and myself down the hall. We sat down and she told me a little bit about the surgery and what to expect. She told me about incision site, the stay in the hospital and the recovery process after. I told the nurse that before she tells me about the surgery that I did *not* wish to know if my heart would be stopped during the surgery. It was a fear of mine that I had and I just didn't want to know the details. Sometimes too much knowledge can instill fear and create the wrong frame of mind or mindset. I wanted to go into surgery with a positive attitude and frame of mind with no fear.

Around 2001, my mother went to Texas to have aorta repair surgery. A few days before the surgery she met with a nurse who explained the surgery to her. The nurse brought a model into the room showing all the internal organs. She sat down and told my mother that first, the kidneys would be removed and placed in a saline solution and would be replaced later. As she said this she plucked the kidneys from the model like she was plucking cherries off of a tree. My mother cringed when she did this and immediately stopped her. My mother told her, "Please don't tell me what the surgeon will do or how he will do it, just do it." This was how I felt before having my surgery. Just do what needs to be done and spare me the details. While some people want to hear all the details, others do not, including myself.

CHAPTER 7

The Surgery and Recovery

The Friday before my surgery my wife, our son and I went out to dinner at a Japanese restaurant for dinner. At first I wanted to stay home, but thought it might be fun and get my mind off the upcoming surgery. When I got to the restaurant the surgery was still at the forefront of my mind. I thought perhaps it would be the last supper for me out at a nice restaurant with my family. Nonetheless, I tried to put my worries on the back burner and enjoy dinner out with my family.

The weekend passed quickly and Monday morning had arrived. I awakened early, showered and prepared for the surgery. Then, I arrived with my wife at the hospital about fifteen minutes before the time I was supposed to check in. After checking in about ten minutes later, a gentleman with a wheel chair came to bring me to a room where body hair would be shaved off and I would be initially prepped for surgery. It was strange because once the time had arrived I was less nervous and more involved in thinking about the process as it would apply to me.

After being shaved, I was wheeled down on my bed to a waiting room with my wife and father who had come to the hospital. About ten minutes later, the anesthesiologist came into the room to explain some details to me. I reminded him about my occasional sleep apnea and my defibrillator and he told me that they were aware of both and not to worry. Then, I was wheeled into surgery. The room was bright and well lit. I remember the anesthesiologist and one other person in the operating room and before I knew it, I was under the anesthetic. When you are under the anesthetic, there is no worry or pain and the experience is transient.

My surgery started at 9am and finished around 11am, but I did not awaken until mid-afternoon. I think perhaps I had slept a bit longer because I was so exhausted from days and nights of worry. Well, at least now I had gotten through the surgery and my recovery was about to begin.

I had a catheter, so I could not use a urinal for a few days. I never had a catheter before and thought perhaps it would be uncomfortable, but it was not. I also had an I.V. in my right arm and a tube which I think was an I.V. in my neck. I also had two chest tubes and a clip attached to my left index finger and I believe an additional external defibrillator was attached to me as a back-up as well. So, I kind of felt like *"The Borg"* from the movie *"Star Trek."*

The first few days I spent in the ICU until I was moved up to my own room. I was feeling good, but my chest incision area hurt. I feel like I sampled every pain pill the hospital had, but nothing seemed to take away the pain. It was funny, because after all the heavy-duty pain medication I was given, the only think that seemed to help a little with the pain was the aspirin Acetaminophen that I take at home. Even though I am not diabetic, I was given insulin in the hospital. I asked the nurse why I needed to be given insulin. She stated that even though I was not diabetic that sometimes the surgery can throw off the insulin levels.

I was also given a spirometer which I used to help keep my lungs healthy after surgery. I started using the device which I was given the week before my surgery. I continued to use it every hour on the hour when I was awake and did so faithfully. After surgery, it may be too painful to take deep breaths in. You may also feel too weak to take deep breaths in. Also, if you do not do deep breathing *after surgery*, you may develop lung problems, like pneumonia. Hence, the use of a spirometer is extremely important to your recovery.

Sleeping when in ICU was much easier than I thought. There is *always* noise and people talking around the clock. However, on the second night that I was in

ICU I was able to sleep through the night. I was fortunate to have outstanding ICU staff assisting me in my recovery. One nurse named Richard was outstanding. He was in my room regularly to check my blood, blood pressure and insulin levels and to give me meds to take. Taking meds was difficult because I had to take my regular meds and also pain pills and supplements like iron. I didn't like the iron pills because they upset my stomach, but my blood was anemic, so I needed to take iron as well as potassium. I just drank lots of water and tried to sit up as much as possible in bed.

Sitting up in bed was difficult, and at times I would slide too far down in my bed and require two staff to yank me back up. I remember the first time I needed assistance being pulled back up. They told me to take a deep breath while they yanked me up back into position. I could feel the pain in my chest and there was lots of pain and discomfort. Also, there were times when I had to be turned and repositioned from one side to the next and the same procedure was used, which caused a bit of pain and discomfort.

As the day was approaching for me to move up to my own private room, a nurse came into my room and told me that she would need to remove my chest tubes, neck tube and catheter. I was so worried about the pain associated with having my catheter and chest tubes removed. However, the nurse was great and talked me through it and told me when to take a deep breath when each chest tube and the catheter tube were being withdrawn. I was always fearful of having a catheter, a breathing tube and open heart surgery, and now it seemed like I had to face all of my fears all at one time. What I learned from the experience was that there are times in our lives when we don't have a choice. When I was told I needed to have open heart surgery I didn't have a choice and time was not a luxury because of the urgency associated with getting the surgery. So, I had no time to get a second opinion. I faced my trials and those things that overwhelmed me squarely and bravely and asked lots and lots of questions along the way before and after the surgery and during my recovery in the hospital and at home and placed myself in God's hands.

Physical therapy came to have me walk the halls as well. Because I was in excellent physical condition both physically and aerobically I did well on my first trial. Being in bed made my muscles weak. So, I was a little wobbly at first, but quickly got grounded and was able to walk with the physical therapist. The physical therapist was impressed. He informed me that once I got up to my own private room that I would walk again with him or with someone else from physical therapy.

Once I was moved up to my own private room from ICU to continue my recovery, I was able to walk with the nurse prior to my physical therapy session. As soon as I was settled in, my wife and my aunt came to visit. I was still experiencing a little discomfort from my chest incision, so I wasn't really up for visitors, but I did my best to be cordial until having to ask them to leave politely so that I could get my rest. My family wanted to stay, but I insisted that I needed to focus inward on myself to heal in mind, body and spirit and get well. I kind of compare this to putting yourself into a mental state or mental frame of mind. Sometimes when you don't feel well you need to have peace and quiet so that you can focus all of your attention and energy on getting well. There are even times when I am driving my vehicle that I shut off the music. I just want to enjoy the peace and the quiet without noise and without distraction.

My family certainly understood and came back the next day. However, my peace and quiet would be short-lived when a patient admitted an hour later a few rooms away from mine would start screaming frantically. The screaming started from late afternoon when she was admitted and continued on into the night. I turned on my television and tried to fall asleep watching television, but to no avail. It was 2am in the morning and I finally called the nurse. I told the nurse that I had worked in a helping profession with people and had infinite patience, tolerance and altruism. However, being a patient myself, I needed my rest also to heal and to get well. I requested a room change. She told me that I wouldn't be able to change rooms, but that she could shut the door to my room. I agreed and was able to fall off to sleep. However, now being in a dark hospital room with the lights off, if I dropped the box which I used to summons assistance or was unable to locate it in the dark, or if I dropped and was unable to find my urinal, then I would be putting myself in jeopardy and even in danger. Nonetheless, I was able to sleep through the night with no issues.

The following day, I did a walk in the morning with the physical therapist. I walked entirely around the hall of the hospital floor that I was on. I walked the length of one hall, stopped, then walked the length of the other hall, stopped and then walked the length of the other connecting hall with no issues. The physical therapist told me that I was ready to go home, but I knew that the cardiac surgeon would make the final determination. Still, I credit my daily exercise routine and treadmill workouts prior to surgery to my success in physical therapy.

My right leg from where the vein was taken was swollen and on the upper-part of my thigh my leg was so swollen that the skin had split open. I was instructed to keep my leg elevated, which I did. The swelling was also in my foot, so I had to wear a loose-fitting pair of sneakers. Even after my discharge from the hospital, I continued to keep my leg elevated for quite a while until the swelling went away.

A little later that day my wife came to visit and at the same time the cardiac surgeon and physician's assistant came to my room. The cardiac surgeon told me that I could go home that morning, or wait until the next day. I didn't think I would survive another day of hospital food, so I expressed my desire to go home that morning. I was admitted on October 9th 2017 and discharged the morning of October 12th. So, not really counting Thursday, I only stayed in the hospital about three days which was extraordinary! The cardiac surgeon told me that the nurse would prepare the discharge papers and then I would be allowed to go home soon after some sutures were removed.

Later, the physician's assistant came into my room and removed some sutures associated with the chest tubes had been removed in the ICU. The removal of the sutures was an agonizing process. The physician's assistant pulled the sutures out a little bit at a time, then a little bit more and a little bit more and a little bit more still. It wasn't too painful, but the sensation of having a suture pulled from your upper-stomach area was not a pleasurable experience to say the least. After pulling out as much suture as she could, she told me she could not remove the rest, and that the remaining sutures would dissolve.

Next, the dietitian who I had requested to speak with came to talk with me. I told her that I was following the dietary program the hospital gave me from when I had my stents in 2013 which included the *healthy* frozen meals. She told me to forget the frozen *healthy* meals and cook my own meals. She also told me to read all labels, count my sodium intake, Trans and saturated fats. She also gave me a book with a diagram which illustrated the breakdown of protein to vegetables to grains on one plate and more. I told her my cholesterol was 98 and triglycerides were 143, but she said that the hereditary factor was strong and that I would be doing the right thing by cooking my own meals, reading labels and counting fats and sodium and keeping my sodium consumption between 1200 - 1500mg daily.

Finally, a nurse came into the room and gave me my discharge papers with post-surgery instructions, instructions about medication and prescriptions to fill. I was also asked if I thought I needed a visiting nurse. Since I had my wife to assist me, I felt I didn't need a visiting nurse to come to my home. After speaking with the nurse, I watched a short discharge video, and then a gentleman with a wheel chair came to bring me down to my wife's car. My father had come to the hospital as well at the time I was being discharged, so we were all able to leave the hospital together.

I remember sitting outside in the wheel chair waiting for my wife to pull up. It was cold and I remember that the outside world looked like I was looking out of a fish bowl. I was just glad to be out of the hospital and finally heading home. When my wife pulled the car up, I was assisted into the car and given the pillow that I was given by the hospital to keep in front of my chest whenever riding in the car until I could drive again to protect my sternum and heart in case of an accident. I positioned it in front of my chest and then fastened my seatbelt and then we proceeded home.

Once I arrived home, my wife helped me out of the car and we proceeded into the house. Even though I was home from the hospital, my recovery was far from over. If anything, my recover was just beginning. The first day home from the hospital all I wanted to do was sleep. I got into bed and I slept. I remember how terrible my stomach felt from not being able to finish the hospital food I was given to eat at the hospital. As a result, after passing a stool the first day that I was home, I was only able to pass clear liquid, and the sensation of having to go came upon me so fast that I had to wear incontinence underwear for men for about a week. I then called my primary care physician and he suggested a laxative which quickly corrected the problem and get my bowels back to normal again.

A number of weeks passed after coming home from the hospital, but my right leg and foot were still swollen. I elevated it when sitting and I elevated it in bed, but could not get the swelling down. I contacted the Doctor's office and asked what I could do. The nurse told me on the phone that I needed to elevate my leg above my heart. This was the mistake that I was making since I was not elevating my leg high enough. As soon as I started elevating my leg more, I slowly started to see the swelling in my leg and foot go down.   All of the swelling had went down except for one pocket of what looked more like fluid retention than swelling behind my right thigh. I immediately contacted my primary care physician who scheduled me for an appointment. Upon examination, he thought it was just residual and told me that it would go away, but that it might take a long time to for everything to return to normal and that I still might feel some numbness in the leg and chest area where the incision was.

Sleeping was also quite a challenge. I was afraid of sleeping flat and on my side because I didn't want to put pressure on my chest as it was still healing. So, I slept in bed slightly elevated, or propped-up. I tried it for a few nights, but it was very uncomfortable. So, I decided to move from the bed to the couch and place a chair in front of me to put my foot on to raise my leg while sleeping upright on the couch with a pillow behind my head. This worked fine for about a week and a half, but soon took its toll on my back. So, I tried sleeping in my bed again and tried both of my regular pillows and a smaller pillow for my head in a different position which finally worked for me.

The second week after my surgery I also started walking. Per the instructions that I received from the hospital, I walked 10 minutes in the morning and 10 minutes in the afternoon. Then, the following week I did 20 minutes in the morning and 20 minutes in the afternoon. Finally, on the third week I was walking from 30 – 40 minutes once a day. I also started some very light and gentle stretching like Thai Chi to keep limber.

A few months into my recovery I also noticed some stinging around the area where my sutures were partially removed and could feel tiny *bumps* under the skin from where the sutures were located. The bumps felt like little pebbles underneath my skin. I was concerned with the stinging and worried that the sutures might cause bleeding, so once again I called my doctor and was told that the sutures would dissolve. I was also told that the sutures raise upwards and not inwards. So, I just to keep an eye in them, but was told that it could take up to 6 months for the sutures to dissolve.

In every instance when I had a question, I called the cardiac surgeon or my primary care physician with any questions that I had concerning my medications, pain, swelling and other concerns. There were times when I felt like maybe I was calling too much, but the office staff encourages patients to call as often as they need to with any and all questions that they may have. So, as I recovered, I was able to get my questions and concerns answered and not feel like I was being a pest. I was made to feel at ease and was given the knowledge I needed to not worry and make progress in my recovery.

CHAPTER 8

Regaining Control of Your Life

After consulting with my cardiologist and the dietitian, I began to understand the reason that I got additional blockages were through no fault of my own. After my heart attack in 2013 and stents, for four years after that I thought I did everything right, and *still* got two blockages for which I needed double bypass surgery. My cardiologist told me that I am fighting the *hereditary factor*, and even though my cholesterol was around 98 and my triglycerides were 143, these numbers in my case didn't tell the whole story of what was truly going on inside me. This is why when my shoulders started to ache during my morning treadmill exercises I went to the emergency room immediately and followed up with a stress test to let the doctor have a look inside me to actually *see* what was going on. By making the decision to have the stress test, the doctor caught the blockages early and I saved my life with bypass surgery, or *"Just in time"* surgery as it has been referred to.

I realized that now I needed to cook my own meals and keep track of my sodium, Trans fats and saturated fat intake. I made the decision to cut out butter, cheese and dairy from my diet, although the dietitian told me I could have butter and cheese once in a while. I still substitute my butter with a butter substitute which I have maybe a few times a month as a treat. I also limit my red meat consumption to once a week. These are all the recommendations that I was told to follow by my doctor and dietitian. However, everyone's case is different, and you should always consult with your own doctor and dietitian so that you can strive to live and eat healthier.

I was more aware now of what I was putting into my mouth, and found substitutes for butter, such as no sugar jams and peanut butter occasionally. I knew now that I had to step-up my game with regard to my diet. When I initially lost 30 pounds back in 2013 after my heart attack I put a plan into action and I was motivated to do so. My plan was to cut out snacks, no more soda (only caffeine-free diet soda and only one-half glass a day) and drink more water and juices. I also went on a low-fat, low sodium diet and ate sugar-free foods as well. Along with a proper diet I worked out on the treadmill 30-36 minutes a day. After a time I started shredding pounds and losing the weight. But now, to fight the hereditary factor I had to do *more.* I had to limit butter and cheese, monitor my sodium, Trans and saturated fats and cook my own meals.

Because of the hereditary factor I had to change the way that I was fighting heart disease. Until I had gained new knowledge, I was just fighting heart disease the way I was instructed to do so by my doctors using information I was given at the hospital at the time of my heart attack in 2013. I knew very little about Trans fats, saturated fats and sodium and the recommended daily allowances for these, and never read the labels on food items. However, after the bypass surgery in 2017, consulting with a dietitian, nurses and my doctor's, this gave me an opportunity to gather new and specialized knowledge to switch lanes and formulate a new battle plan for fighting heart disease and the hereditary factor. Sometimes, we can set a course in life that does not work out or does not meet our expectations. We can, however, switch lanes and choose a different course. While it is not always easy to switch lanes in life and choose a new course, it is possible. When we choose to switch lanes, we do so because we feel that we can do better and improve the present condition of our lives. In some cases, switching lanes will improve ones' life, but in other cases the new situation we may find ourselves in may actually be worse or not make a difference at all. When I was in the hospital, I told the nurse that I wanted to speak to a dietitian, and she told me that, "Even though you may change your diet, it may not make a difference." I told her that regardless, I was still going to try. While her statement seemed kind of cold and lacking empathy, perhaps it was something that I had needed to hear. The hereditary factor is a fierce adversary, and keeps you on your toes when you have heart disease to eat right and exercise.

You have to remember that with heart disease, involvement and education are so important. Ask questions, go to lectures, take exercise classes and invest in yourself and improve your health and your life. If you smoke, all the more reason to take control of your life is to kick an annoying habit. Perhaps you are addicted to smoking or drinking for instance. These are not hobbies or pass times, these are vices, and each taken to excess can rob us of our health and have the potential to ruin our lives. Smoking can destroy our health and our lives and is detrimental to those with heart disease, not to mention the cost of cigarettes and the impact that smoking has on our wallets and our pocketbooks. Some might try to kick this habit on their own, find support groups or go to a doctor or hypnotherapist to try to stop smoking. You should be comfortable with the method you choose to quit smoking and not get discouraged if you don't succeed the first time.

To truly take control of our lives and combat heart disease and the hereditary factor, we must be willing to change so that we feel strong, vibrant and alive on the inside so that we can master our destiny, our health and our lives. To do this, we must strive to achieve optimum health. When I wake each morning, I literally exercise my way out of bed. I start with stretching exercises for the back while in bed, and then sit on the edge of the bed and exercise the ankles, toes and extend the legs to get my circulation going, and then do some yoga stretching for each part of my body to start the day or Thai Chi. I do aerobics 30 - 36 minutes a day of aerobics and eat healthy foods and consume healthy drinks while limiting salt and sugar and cut out snacks by substituting fruits and eat lots of vegetables. These are the things I do each day for optimum health so that I can better control my life and my health. Like me, you can find things that work well for you too!

Heart disease, like any kind of disease, can bring us down and affect our mind, body and spirit. We need to gather our forces and achieve balance in these areas. Fighting the hereditary factor means following a very strict diet, and eating a certain way and buying all the things I need to eat a diet low in trans fats, low in saturated fat and low in sodium can cost money, lots of money. This, in turn, can place a strain on the family budget. Food stamps and state assistance can help as well as budgeting each month. Once you have established a diet you can get an idea of how much you will need to spend each month in order to purchase the foods you require to maintain your diet.

Sticking to that diet can be difficult. Too many times I was tempted by sweet treats and needed to reinforce my new behaviors with positive self-talk and daily affirmations. I'm sure you've heard the saying, "We are what we eat"? Well, we can also substitute the word *think* for eat; hence: we are what we think! Positive daily self-talk is so important, because like the use of auto suggestion in hypnosis, through positive daily affirmations we are directing our minds in a positive direction by nurturing our subconscious mind with positive thoughts and affirmations which help strengthen our minds and condition our thought patterns to attune to the goals and objectives we set for ourselves in life. For instance, we can write out a particular affirmation that we can say each morning upon awakening. Here is an example.

AFFIRMATION FOR WELLNESS: The wellspring that flows in and through my body and my mind at this very moment is giving me strength, vitality, energy and power and wellness and making me feel vibrant, alive, young, vital and powerful; making me feel better every day in every way.   I now send these thoughts and feelings to every part of my body to revitalize my cells in my body, my heart and my mind: I am power, I am strength, I am vital, I am alive, I am vibrant, I am well!

To fight the hereditary factor we may have to change our methods if what we are doing is not succeeding. This often means changing ourselves which means being willing to make sacrifices. Being willing to give up and limit certain foods for instance and make the dietary and life changes necessary to succeed under the advice of your doctor and dietitian. Many of my friends who have heart disease have returned to their old ways. One of my friends lifts heavy objects, shovels, mows the lawn and eats fast foods. Another person once told me that he will eat anything he wants because it takes years for arteries to re-clog. If I lived my life like either of these people, I might not be here now. Listen to and follow the advice of your doctor's and dietitian, get checkups and stress tests and if something doesn't feel quite right, don't hesitate and go immediately to the emergency room. Prevention saves lives and *prevention* and *knowledge* are powerful allies in fighting heart disease and the hereditary factor.

About the Author

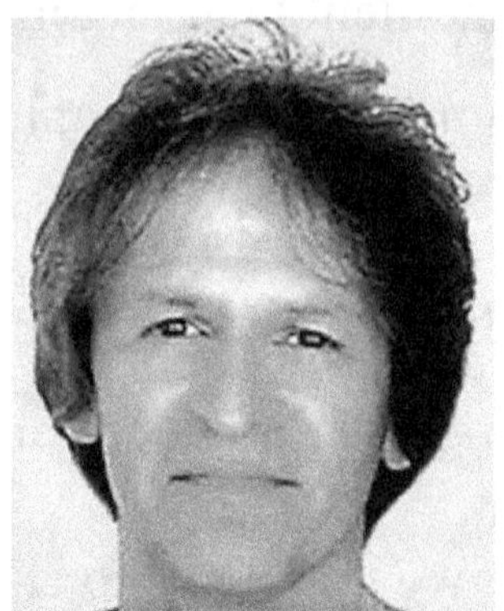

David James Zoppi is an author and writer of stories and short-stories. David also holds a master's degree in rehabilitation counseling, is a certified health coach and has a Ph.D. in business. David has devoted his life to helping people throughout his life and imparts his knowledge and wisdom to help others.